This notebook belongs to:

....

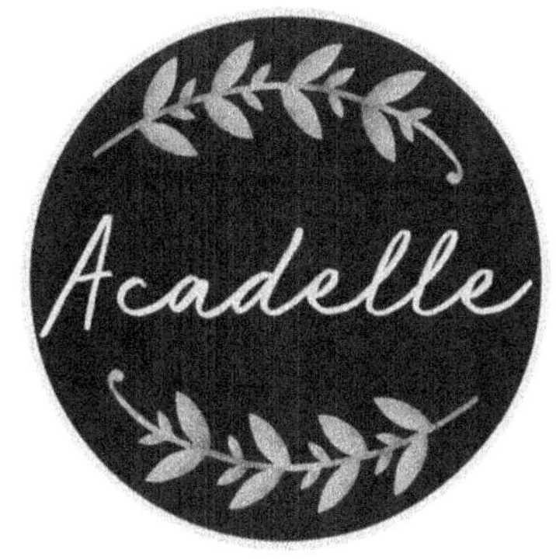

Visit us at www.acadelle.com for more notebooks, planners and other awesome vegan goodies.

Follow us on Facebook: facebook.com/acadelle

Friends Not Food

www.ingramcontent.com/pod-product-compliance
Lightning Source LLC
Chambersburg PA
CBHW081618250726
48657CB00009B/2616